A Dy

A Helen Arkell Dyslexia Charity Publication

An Introduction to Dyslexia, A Dyslexic's Eye View
Author Helen Arkell
Published by The Helen Arkell Dyslexia Charity
24 West Street, Farnham, Surrey, GU9 7DR

First Published 1973
Reprinted 1990 & 1997
Revised Edition 2023

Printed in England by Kall Kwik Farnham

The Helen Arkell Dyslexia Charity
A Company limited by guarantee. Registered in England Number 3432423
Registered Charity Number 1064646

FOREWORD

In this introduction to dyslexia (specific learning difficulty) I am trying, as a dyslexic, to explain in simple language what it is like if you have this problem. It can be extremely difficult for a parent or teacher to understand why their bright child persists in making apparently elementary mistakes.

Although it is many years since I first tried to describe this condition, and much has evolved in the field of recognition and remediation since then, the basic difficulties and the feelings of the individual remain exactly the same.

Helen Arkell
Frensham 1997

When we rediscovered this little gem of a book in autumn 2018, we read it through to see how much needed to be changed and very little did. Helen's words are as relevant today as when they were first written.

Yvonne Whitestone
Head of Education

The Author

Helen Arkell was herself dyslexic and had a deep understanding of the many ways dyslexia can affect people. She knew what it was like to feel different, to be regarded as stupid when you know inside you are not, and appreciated the fears that parents of dyslexic children have. She also felt strongly that dyslexia is not to be feared because it can be a positive force. Dyslexics have many valuable talents and can achieve as much as anyone else.

After training in Denmark, she started teaching dyslexic children at her home during the early 1960's when dyslexia was unrecognised and disregarded, and was probably the first person in this country to provide such help. She also taught at the Word Blind Centre in Coram Fields, London, until that closed in the late 1960's.

Fearing that the awareness of dyslexia that had started to develop would die out and nothing more would be done to help dyslexic people, she bought a house in Fulham Road, London. With the help of Joy Pollock and Elizabeth Waller, she opened the Helen Arkell Dyslexia Centre in April 1971 – both there and at her home in Frensham, Surrey. The Charity is now based in Farnham and has become one of the country's leading dyslexia organisations.

Helen received an MBE in 1999 for her work in dyslexia and further royal recognition followed in 2003 when she was honoured as a Pioneer to the Life of the Nation at a Buckingham Palace reception.

Contents

For the purpose of clarity, the child is referred to as 'he' and the teacher as 'she'.

Introduction

"I know words and how to talk because I know what words mean in my life, but reading isn't in my life at all."

This was said to me by a nine year old boy.

How did you learn to read?

Was it difficult?

How old were you when you could read?

To the average person these simple questions do not seem threatening but for anyone for whom learning to read has been an uphill and often traumatic experience it is a different matter.

In this short introduction to the problem of dyslexia, I am trying to explain to the person who is not dyslexic, in simple terms, what it is like to be dyslexic, and what sort of problems it brings in its wake.

In my thirty years as a remedial teacher, my own dyslexia has been a help to me because it has made it easier for me to understand the difficulties of my pupils. When I quote from their experiences and from my own, it is in the hope of showing the reader how the effect on the individual may reach far beyond the actual problem of poor reading and spelling.

This condition has no outward symptoms and, because the sufferer is normal in other things, it is often wrongly diagnosed and misunderstood.

Then, to add to a child's worries, he may be labelled lazy and careless: he may be accused of not trying and the comment 'could do better' or 'must try harder' is likely to appear on his reports with monotonous regularity.

Those who have learned to read and spell with comparative ease during their first years at school will find it difficult to understand why something that they have assimilated without conscious effort could be such a mammoth task for others. They will probably not stop to think about what complex processes are involved in acquiring and using the skills which deal with the decoding of symbols in reading, and with the encoding of the spoken word in the case of writing.

In our society words are used – squandered one might say – incessantly. Spoken words are heard constantly – our families and friends, our neighbours, voices on the radio or on television speaking directly to us or as a background sound. Endless words are written and read; many simple events in everyday life are dependent on the individual being able to read and write. Much information is gained from letters, books and newspapers. Instructions and announcements need to be read and the person who cannot read warning notices may be in physical danger.

Messages and instructions need to be written, and numerous forms must be filled in for a variety of reasons. Those who have not acquired the necessary skills to deal with written language will be under a severe handicap; they will miss important information, they may easily be cheated, they are likely to have a grave feeling of inferiority and they will probably be looked down upon by their more fortunate peers.

One of our adult pupils had saved enough money and found the courage to take her small daughter to Greece for a holiday. She had taken every precaution she could think of to ensure that she would not have to read or write. She had the luggage labels for her return journey with her, as well as some postcards to friends saying that she was having a nice time. Everything went smoothly, and in the coach taking her to the airport for her return journey she was thinking how much she had enjoyed it all, and at no time had she been in danger of having her secret found out. On arrival at the airport all the passengers were handed a form to fill in relating to their nationality, passport number, etc. Her description of the panic that seized her was heartbreaking. I do not know what ultimately went down on the form but she arrived back in a highly emotional state and with a bitter sense of failure.

People who are weak in other areas do not suffer the same indignities. Some, for example, are totally unable to sing in tune, or indeed, to tell one note from another; they are not labelled lazy or thick. Some cannot distinguish certain colours; this presents some practical problems, but their peers do not think of them as stupid or uneducated. Some have little or no control over their body movements so they are never chosen on team games; some cannot screw a screw in straight but they are not taunted and accused of being backward.

In any book or any lecture on dyslexia the word *perception* is bound to be mentioned, and it is worth considering the literal meaning. A dictionary will define it something like this: 'Recognition with understanding' or 'Faculty by which man has knowledge through the medium of the bodily organs'. So the senses through which we see, hear, smell, taste, and feel give us the information but the meaning of this information has to be processed in the brain. You may see a written text but unless it is understood there is no perception. It is in the processing of material represented by symbols that a dyslexic's main problem lies. However, recognising symbolic material tends to be easier than writing it and it is not uncommon to find a child, or indeed an adult, who has overcome his problem with reading, but who still has enormous problems with spelling. There are a few whose spelling is ahead of their reading, although this is unusual.

The problems touched on above relate largely to poor perception, but these will not be the only ones. Some difficulty with sequencing and orientation is almost certainly experienced and often there has been a delay in acquiring speech, as well as in the motor control required for certain skills.

The relative strengths and weaknesses will vary from child to child. It is important for a teacher to be able to identify the reason for underachievement, so I am attempting to list some of the common symptoms under relevant chapters. However, any one group should not be thought of in isolation because the child's difficulties will relate to several, if not all, of the chapters. Each chapter should be seen as merely one aspect of the whole problem.

Poor Visual Perception

Poor visual perception has nothing to do with any eye problems that may be present but, as already suggested, it is a difficulty in associating the symbol seen with the sound it represents. The child will be slow in taking in a whole word in such a way that he will recognise it when he sees it again. He will then be unable to recall the look of it when he wants to write it. Most people carry a picture of a word in their mind's eye – how long it is, the general outline, its main features – but the child with poor visual perception will have only a vague, or in some cases virtually no recollection of the look of a word. If you write it on a blackboard he will see it as clearly as anyone else, but when you rub it out it is as though it has been erased from his mind. One could say that poor visual perception is the opposite of a photographic memory.

The child may struggle to read a word on one line and, when he sees the same word on the next line, he will look at it as though he has never seen it before. Many people, if they are in doubt about the spelling of a word, may write it down in two or three ways, and they can see which one is right, but if you cannot recall what the word should look like you will not easily be able to spot which one is correct. Often a pupil will write a word, perhaps with help from the teacher, and having finished it look at it in surprise and say, **"Oh, I thought it was going to be much longer!"** or some other remark, which shows that when he started to write it he had no idea what the end product was going to look like.

If these children are distracted when reading – even momentarily – it is interesting to note that they cannot find the place where they left off. Other people seem able to go straight back, but those with poor visual recall will have forgotten the layout of the page and where they were in relation to a full stop or paragraph; they may even have forgotten whether they were on the right or

left hand page and they will waste time reading a few lines here and a few lines there in search of
their place.

I sometimes ask pupils whether they experience this difficulty and frequently the answer is **"No, that's no problem, because whenever I look away I put my thumb at the end of the line I'm on."** Their answer, of course, should not be that they have no problem, but that they have found an effective way of coping with it.

It follows that copying from the blackboard is a worrying task. The child who cannot hold the visual pattern of a word or words in his mind's eye will have to look at the board many more times than his peers. As he works along the line he will find it increasingly difficult to identify the place he has reached and, if there are several lines, his predicament will be worse. He is lucky if he has copied half the passage by the time the class has finished. Either it will be rubbed off or a kindly teacher will hold up the class to wait for him. In either case he feels under intolerable pressure and, after a few experiences of this nature, tension and anxiety will build up even before he starts to write; and so a further problem is added to the picture.

Sometimes a child may tell you that the letters on a page will not keep still. In that case an orthoptist should be consulted.

The example that follows is an extract from dyslexic scuba diver, an old friend of mine, who was pretty sound phonetically but who had not got the visual recall to spot his mistakes.

I'v hadsum grate dive a round
Sydney, when everything is in you
Paver. water condition s, viserbitatey,
marine liPe & diving lokeashon.

Poor Auditory Perception

The child who is weak auditorily is likely to have been slow in learning to speak, and he has probably gone on talking baby language longer than the average child. There is no actual speech defect, but he will often continue to mispronounce words because he is not aware of the exact sounds within them. He will probably have poor discrimination and be confused between sounds that are similar, such as *d* and *t* or *m* and *n.* Short vowels nearly always cause difficulties. They have little character and, as one boy put it, in isolation they are *"just a series of grunts"*. The child with this type of difficulty may not be able to tap out a rhythm. When speaking he may put the emphasis on the wrong syllables or get the wrong number of syllables in a word. He may say *"unimous"* or *"unaninimous"* instead of *"unanimous".* Often he has difficulty in finding a rhyming word. He may be bad at blending sounds when reading; although he can say the sounds *m-a-n* he cannot necessarily blend the sounds into the word *man.* Conversely, if you put the letters *m, a* and *n* in front of him and say "this says man, what will it say if I take the *m* away?", he will be unable to isolate the sounds in such a way that he can give the answer. Pronunciation of words may be muddled. He may say his mother has gone to "hostipal", or that he enjoyed his holiday looking at "the Roman merains". The correct sounds are all in the words, but the order is wrong. He will be slow to learn a new word and, even when he seems to have grasped it and used it correctly for some time, he may for no apparent reason use it in the wrong context or substitute it for a word which sounds similar.

He may have been taught to read by the whole word method – the look and say – or, he may have found through experience that although his visual recall is weak, it serves him better than his auditory recall. So this child will try to rely on his visual recall and remember what letters were in a word or what the whole word looks like. He may write "evnelope". He has memorised the letters in the word but his visual recall is not accurate enough for him to see that the order of the letters is not correct. He does not work phonetically through the sounds so he cannot tell through the auditory channel that there is a transposal.

He may write the word **bely** instead of **help.** In this case he is trying to remember the general outline of the word.

Learning foreign languages is usually a stumbling block and many experts recommend that they should be avoided – at least the written word – until the child has mastered his mother tongue.

Kinaesthetic Approach in Writing

Learning to write is a long and arduous for any child, but by degrees he will learn to write certain words without conscious effort. He will start no doubt with his own first name. As time goes by and he progresses up the school, he will acquire an increasingly large vocabulary of words that his hand will write almost automatically without having to think about it in detail.

A dyslexic may be slow to acquire the *feel* of the written word. Unless he is concentrating on the movement of the tip of his pen all the time, it will acquire a will of its own and make a spelling mistake or write the wrong word altogether. To illustrate this I mention my own difficulty to this day in writing a word containing a double m – I have to count the loops as I go or I will get the wrong number. In the same way a dyslexic child will have to keep reminding himself that the letter i must be dotted and the t crossed. It does not become an automatic action and he is just as likely to cross his i's instead. A young woman described it as follows – **"Every time I write something my brain has a fight with my hand and my hand often wins".**

If your main attention is on the tip of your pen you easily lose the context of what you are writing and forget the good sentence you had planned. You may forget that you are writing in the past tense and switch to the present or you may go from the third person to the first or lose the flow of your sentence.

If a child cannot remember the look of a word, if he cannot easily sort out the sounds within a word, if he cannot help himself by the feel of writing a word, each word that he learns to spell becomes a feat of memory; but memorising the right letters in words is not enough, they have to be in the correct order or sequence or he may write *on* for *no, who* for *how, left* for *felt,* and this brings me to the next problem.

Sequencing

Sequencing in any form may be difficult for a dyslexic child. He may know the names of the letters of the alphabet, but have difficulty in memorising the correct order.

Having learnt the order he will not automatically know where one letter comes in relation to another. If you ask "Which comes first, *k* or *t?"* he will probably not know nor will he have any idea whether they are close in the alphabet or whether there are many letters between them. He will have to go back to the beginning of the alphabet and go right through the sequence to see which comes first and how far it is to the next one. It does not take much imagination to appreciate what this child will feel like when the teacher says, "For homework look up the following ten words in the dictionary."

Learning the order of the days of the week and the months of the year may be equally hard, or it may be the letters within a word, or the sequence of events either in his own life or in history.

Many of my pupils have heard the anecdote about the annoyance I felt one evening on coming across a sign saying *auction* just by some road works. A few days later, taking the same road, I found that the sign did not say *auction* but *caution.*

A boy told me about an exciting war film he had seen called *The Battle of the Bugle;* the story content seemed familiar and eventually I realised he was talking about *The Battle of the Bulge*.

A child may change the order of words in sentence. You may dictate to him *"He was too dreamy"* and he will write *"He too was dreamy".* The correct words are all in the sentence, but the sense has been changed slightly. You may give some instructions to a child – "Go indoors, take off your boots, then go upstairs and wash your hands". A double problem will arise here. With poor short term memory (see chapter on Short Term Memory), and sequencing problems, the child may remember some of the main points but forget others and, confusing the order of events , be found upstairs washing his gum boots in the basin.

It is important for parents and teachers alike to understand that there can be real misunderstandings over instructions if they contain several separate activities.

Orientation

Any young child will find it difficult to remember which is his right hand and which is his left. Initially he will probably find some mnemonic to help him, like a scar on one hand or, if he is right handed, he may remember that he writes with his right hand. By degrees the knowledge of which hand is which becomes automatic with most children, but this is not necessarily so for the dyslexic. He may have to rely on his mnemonic all his life and, while he will become increasingly quick at working it out, a situation in which he feels under pressure may see him react incorrectly. A large number of soldiers on parade grounds who turn wrongly to left or right have been found to have reading and spelling problems.

There may be other directional confusions such as *in* and *out, up* and *down.* When writing the child may write the letter d instead of g or vice versa. The shapes are the same to start with and when it comes to deciding whether the long stroke should go up or down he has no automatic feeling for which way it should go. When trying to write the letter he may do the initial c shape, then go round and round trying to decide at which side he should finish it.

Learning North, South, East and West is particularly difficult because the points of the compass cannot be learned related to himself; they depend on which way he is facing. Even after grasping the broad principles he may find it hard to understand that France is south of Britain but north of Italy.

One woman gave me a graphic description of her need for time to work out the points of the compass, despite her intellectual understanding of them. "If I want to understand the weather forecast and what weather is expected in various regions I have to mentally prepare myself. I have to drop what I am doing and visualise the map of northern Europe. I imagine myself standing in southern England and looking towards Scotland. Then I know that the Americas are round on the left and that Scandinavia is a bit up on the right. I sort out which is North, South, West and East. Thus organised I can take in the forecast but without it, although I understand every word, I have not understood the meaning".

The child who does not easily understand spatial relationships when they are represented by symbols will probably be slow in learning to tell the time. The difficulties he has are much the same as any child will have in the early stage, but his will persist long after the average child has grasped how to read the clock. Which way round do the hands go? Why does the small hand tell the big hours and the big hand the small minutes? Which side is to the hour and which side is past? All these items of information must be learned and their interdependence understood. In some miraculous way the average child's inbuilt computer manages in time to interrelate all these facts and reach the right answer, but the child to whom such associations do not come readily is under a severe handicap and, at the time when the class is ready to move on to other things, he may still be struggling to remember which side is *to* and which is *past* the hour. At some stage this inability to tell the time will become an embarrassment to him. He will arrive either late or too early for school or for appointments and each time may be forced into a lot of excuses and fibs to try and explain away his mistakes.

Whether the advent of the digital watch is an advantage in this context is open for debate.

Sometimes pupils have not remembered which side of a page to rule the margin: or, if the margin was too broad, on which side of it they were to write.

In the learning of many of the time/space/number concepts which are represented by symbols there may be a double difficulty. If a child is told to rule a margin on the left of his paper he may not remember which side the word left represents. Secondly unlike his peers, he may have failed to get the automatic feel of which side a margin should go even when he has done it many times. Many will be unable to write a column of words or figures neatly below one another, and this will obviously cause great confusion in number work.

Tying shoelaces becomes second nature to most people, but this is a task requiring both spatial and sequencing skills. With which hand does one make the initial loop? Which way round does the other lace go? At which point does one poke it through to form the second loop? The reader would probably be surprised to know how many people wear slip on shoes for the simple reason that they cannot tie shoelaces satisfactorily.

A dyslexic may have a good sense of shape so he will see that a b,d, p and q are the same shape. What is hard for him to remember is in which position does this shape make what sound. Further complications can arise because the capital D has its “bulge” on the right, the lower case on the left. In the letter p, the capital and lower case are much the same shape and it is the size and positioning that are important. Simon was confused by this.

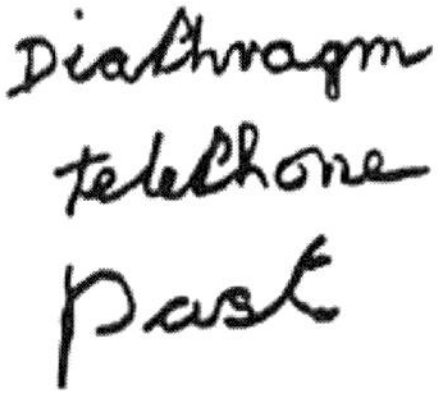

Some children who have this syndrome are delighted to find that they can read equally well with the book upside down. Others can read mirror writing and some can write it without any more effort than ordinary writing.

Short Term Memory

Research is in progress in many countries into the working of the memory, the difference between the short term and the long term memory, and how information gets from one to the other. Suffice it to say here that most people with specific learning difficulty have difficulty in holding verbal information in the short term memory. The saying "in one ear and out the other" is very descriptive of this condition.

A child may be given a dictation, "A dog chased the cat into the wood". The sentence itself may be quickly forgotten though the action may have been understood and the child may write, "A dog ran after the cat into the wood".

A parent may say "Please go to the Post Office and buy a first class stamp for this letter and post it". The maddening reply may come back, "Where shall I take the letter?" The child has genuinely forgotten the beginning of the sentence before the end has been reached. Many people will feel that all children do this but the unretentive short term memory is different from the slightly scatterbrained child who is not paying attention. Again I quote a former pupil, aged nine this time, "**My memory isn't working well today. I'll have to use my brain instead".**

Once information has been fully assimilated it will be retained but it may take keen observation by any teacher involved to locate in which areas the problems lie and it may need imagination and a lot of overlearning to rectify.

Word Retrieval

A tantalising aspect of dyslexia experienced by some sufferers – and one which bothered me considerably – is the difficulty in finding the word one wants at the moment it is needed. This has been referred to as poor word retrieval. Although it may sometimes be experienced by non-dyslexics, I am speaking here about a persistent condition.

A young child may want to relate an event in his day or the story of a television programme he has seen. There will be lots of 'ums' and 'ahs', he will fiddle with his buttons or wriggle in his chair and whatever information he succeeds in producing will come out in a slow disjointed way. He has the vocabulary he needs and he knows what he wants to say but he seems unable to find the words needed to produce an organised sentence. It is as though his vocabulary is badly filed so that he is searching through his system against time instead of the necessary word popping up automatically.

Children have a way of hitting the nail on the head. Tim was no exception although he was not yet eight at the time. **"I can think all right,"** he said. **"What is wrong is just my words."** When writing there is more time to organise one's thoughts and sentences, but even familiar words may be elusive just when they are wanted, though they readily come to mind at other times.

As with so many problems, it is largely up to the individual to find a way of circumventing an obstacle. I became aware that many of my pupils had found the same partial solutions that I had employed myself. As soon as we had been given a subject to write about – maybe days before we had really started to work on it – we would jot down on a piece of paper words that we were likely to need, as they come to mind. This would save us time and avoid frustration. We agreed that a dictionary of synonyms is especially useful for looking up a word with a similar meaning, we might find the exact one we wanted.

I have described the above in some detail to try to make the reader understand what a laborious task it can be to manage just one aspect of specific learning difficulty.

Other Symbols

When we speak of dyslexia we refer to the difficulty of manipulating and understanding letters in reading and writing. Similar problems may be experienced in interpreting other symbols. The child may have difficulty in relating the correct quantity to a given number. He will persist in mirror writing some figures long after most children have learned the correct way. He may write 74 when he means 47 or read 1397 when it should be 1937. When writing a column of figures he may not understand where the units, tens and hundreds should go. The principles behind adding, subtracting, multiplying and dividing may not be readily understood and a confusing factor is introduced in that the child has been constantly told to work from left to right in reading and writing and now, faced with certain sums, he must suddenly work from right to left.

All these problems I have experienced and mostly overcome, but one stubborn hurdle will, I feel sure, be with me always and I share this with most of my fellow sufferers, even those who are good at mathematics; it is the inability to learn tables.

Another thorn in my flesh is dialling telephone numbers. When I tell my friends that I first dialled a wrong number it is easy for them to laugh and say that it is lack of concentration. They may be right that I should concentrate harder, but then they do not have to give their full and undivided attention to obtaining a telephone number, covering each digit as it has been dialled for fear that it might slip in again later or change places with one that has yet to come.

Reading music may equally present a problem. Though the child may be musical he may not be able to understand the association between the written music and the notes he has to play. If he is learning the piano he must read not only one line but two simultaneously, and each hand must follow the correct line. There may be a series of notes going down on the music, which is in an upright position in from of him, but he must interpret whether down is to the right or to the left on the keyboard which is flat.

Punctuation is another obstacle when its use fails to become automatic, sometimes even after bizarre spelling has been rectified. A dyslexic will probably omit it altogether or else put signs at random without really understanding their purpose. A young man I used to teach had three 'A' levels, but he failed the English 'O' level examination several times. His essays were long and interesting although his spelling was unorthodox but his punctuation seemed non-existent. I made some light-hearted remark about the latter being conspicuous by its absence, at which he looked rather hurt and asked whether I had not noticed that he always put a full stop at the bottom of each page!

Although a person with a specific reading difficulty may have learned the rules of punctuation, he may find them difficult to apply. He seems unaware that a comma, a question mark or inverted commas are both necessary and important parts of a sentence.

It can be seen that interpreting symbols is the basis of the dyslexic's problem – symbols which are letters, punctuation, numbers, dots and dashes for morse code, musical notes – any of these may cause confusion.

Motor Control and Handwriting

Many experts find that dyslexic children are clumsy. While this is sometimes evident, there are other cases where the term, as used by the layman, would not apply. Some are excellent games players, or good at making models. Some make intricate constructions with Lego or manage complex games on a computer. Many go on to become good mechanics, engineers and architects or distinguished doctors, surgeons or dentists. They will probably have difficulty getting the necessary qualifications, but once this hurdle is behind them they may have exceptional ability in their chosen field.

In contrast to the ability of many to cope with manipulative tasks the same people will find the process of writing difficult and good clear handwriting is rarely found among children with specific learning difficulty. Their letters are often ill formed and mis-shapen, sometimes to the point of being unrecognisable.

The slope of the writing may change each time a pupil starts a fresh piece of work or, indeed, the letters within a single word may slope at differing angles. A generally spiky appearance is characteristic and the overall impression is untidy and messy, with words crossed out and attempted a second or third time. The capitals may be left out or in the wrong places; they, and the lower case letters may be much the same size and neither placed in the line, but wandering vaguely a bit above or below it. At the top of the following page is the writing of an intelligent ten year old.

Difficulty in performing certain actions requiring complex co-ordination is noted in many dyslexic children, even those who are competent at manipulative tasks. Many of them never crawled as babies and slowness seems to be experienced in learning to swim or ride a bicycle. I bear the scars to this day from my early disasters on a bicycle.

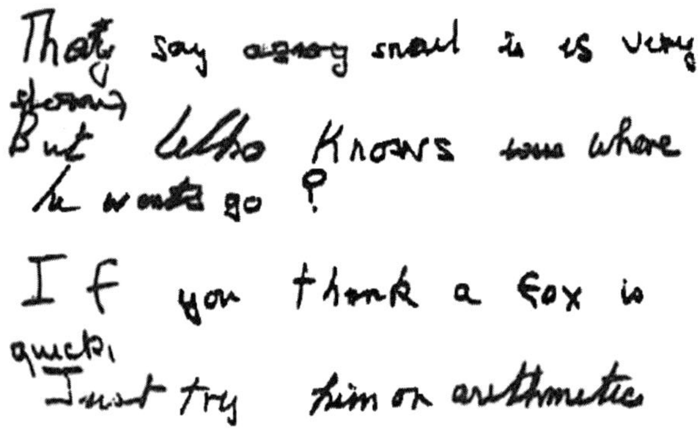

(Examples of handwriting referred to on the previous page.)

How is it that someone who is not sure which side of a page to draw the margin can visualise and draw a complex building?

How is it that someone who can manipulate delicate and minute pieces of machinery is unable to guide his pen across the paper to produce acceptable handwriting?

How is it that a man who failed to get into the Zurich Polytech could develop the Theory of Relativity? Yes, Einstein was dyslexic.

These are just a few of the anomalies found within the dyslexic population. I offer no explanations. I merely state the fact.

The Emotional Effect

A picture of dyslexia would be incomplete without some mention of the emotional effect.

Any child of normal intelligence will become uneasy and in due course worried when he realises that he is being left behind by the rest of the class in almost all subjects. He may become aware quite early on that he is somehow different and inadequate. He cannot analyse this as anxiety but he may start to lose confidence.

The more intelligent child will be in a better position to find ways around his difficulty but is also likely to suffer from greater frustration or worry if he does not succeed. The effect on a child and the time when emotional problems start to build up depend on a variety of factors. The main ones are the degree of the dyslexia, the intelligence and the temperament of the child and the attitude to his problems in the home and at the school.

Different children will react in different ways. One child may have temper tantrums and nightmares. Another may find that the best policy is never to draw attention to himself in the classroom in the hope of being overlooked; he may sit dreaming of other things, losing his ability to concentrate and his interest in learning. Others try to draw attention to themselves and become disruptive in lessons or violent in the playground. Some who have been laughed at for their mistakes, which are frequently very funny, find that the best way to avoid ridicule is to join in the fun, pretend it was all on purpose and a joke. Then they get accepted, often with fondness, as the class buffoon. Some may become increasingly anxious about school and finally refuse to go altogether.

One young man I used to teach had twice been to a young offenders' institution. As I got to know him, I was able to piece together some of the events of his past. He did very badly at his primary school, so his parents sent him to a private school with small classes thinking this would solve everything. However, he was soon labelled thick and was teased for his mistakes by his classmates. Then he found that he could buy peace by bribing the boys to leave him alone. Inevitably his pocket money ran out so he went to the pockets of others to keep up the supply of bribes. He was found out and expelled from the school, but the same sequence of events was repeated at another school, and another. As time went on his tormentors expected larger bribes and he turned to shoplifting. If this young man had been given a little of the right help at the right time it is probable that none of these complications would have followed.

It gives food for thought that some of the many illiterates who are found in our prisons may have got there directly or indirectly as a result of a specific learning difficulty having been neglected.

It is no exaggeration to say that the emotional problems that can arise on account of dyslexia may be far more damaging to an individual than the dyslexia itself. Some people can get on well despite deplorable spelling and inadequate reading as long as they have the confidence to 'bash on'. But once a person's confidence has been undermined, he will become hesitant in all things and come to expect failure.

Some robust personalities succeed despite their problems. Others take knocks during their schooling, but do well once they are not hemmed in by the very thing they are worst at – interpreting symbols. Many of us have been surprised to learn that an old schoolfriend who was thought to be stupid at school has done well in some field. Nelson Rockefeller did not do badly! Lloyd George got round his reading difficulty by having someone to give him a synopsis of the many papers he had to deal with. Susan Hampshire rose to fame almost because of her dyslexia – she was determined to succeed at something.

The following describes what one young woman felt about her education:

My Education

When I frist went to school I played with toys for thefirst week. Then they took away the toys, and gave me pencil and paper, the Teacher wrote a, b, c, The ABC just did not mean a thing to me. I think that if they had keept the toys And if you saw doll, to look at the teacher, would say the word and put the word beside the doll
Next I went into the junior school, haveing hated every moment of the Infant School In a world full of words books, tears
The teacher would say Lynne, stand up and tell me what is the word I have writen on the board' I can tell you It did not mean a think to me, The Class would laugh because I did not reply and the teacher would get very angry. If only she knew what I feelt inside, she would have never made me go through it why she did not set the Class a story to read or write, and taken me or a few others to one side, and looked at how we put down letters, she would soon see that I was not day dreaming. that words, just did not seem to make any kind of sense Well belive it or not I went to my Secondary School knowing very little of English. Well I hated this School, Even my head mistress said to me why Lynne when I ask you a question can you anser it, but when you put it down on paper it never makes sense How on earth could I anser that one I only hope that it never happend to any one else to go through school with so much to say, but with No Key to open the door!

Lynne looks back on her education as a long, unhappy experience although she gradually overcame most of her spelling difficulties and acquired a clear handwriting. How then must a man or woman feel who has left school semi or indeed totally illiterate?

> Many dare not go to a Job Centre for fear of being asked to fill in a form.
>
> Others are in menial jobs despite superior intelligence.
>
> Some refuse promotion because it might involve them in more reading or spelling.
>
> One man always carried an empty spectacle case in his pocket so he could say he had forgotten his glasses if called upon to read or write.
>
> One girl refused all dinner dates because she could not read a menu.

It is never too late to help an adult both with his literacy inadequacies and with the emotional problems that have ensued. However, not many admit to their dilemma. Thanks to the lack of help in school and lack of understanding in the community they feel too ashamed to come forward.

How to Spot the Dyslexic

If parents are aware that their child's progress is slower than his peers in the early stages of learning they should discuss it with the class teacher and also with the head teacher. It may be suggested that, as a first step, the child's eyesight and hearing should be tested. If there is nothing unusual in these areas, parents, in discussion with school, may consider an assessment. The results will show whether your child is performing to his ability level and if not where his weaknesses lie and also his strengths.

If, as a result of tests, your child is said to have dyslexia (or a specific learning difficulty) it often comes as a relief to parents who know that it will respond to specialist teaching.

The number of children who are underachieving is sufficient to warrant the attention of both class teachers and specialist teachers. The interest among teachers is growing and so is the number of courses available to them.

The assessment should be explained to the child in words suited to his age. He must be told that his lack of success at school is not due to poor intelligence nor is it because he is lazy. He has a weakness which means he does not learn reading and writing as easily as other children. However, he may be much better than them at other things. He must also be told that he will need both courage and perseverance and a lot of hard work to overcome it, but with help and understanding from school, support and guidance from home and his own persistent efforts, the handicap will slowly start to recede and eventually be surmounted.

Parents often report a striking change in their child during the first few weeks he is having specialist teaching. This is obviously not so much due to what he has learned in so short a time, but more to the fact that his problem is now understood by himself and by others and that steps are being taken to deal with it.

If a parent or a teacher is wondering what to look for, the following list of possible symptoms may be of help. They are mistakes that any child will make in the initial stages of his learning, but if they persist beyond the time most children have grown out of them, they may indicate dyslexia. It must be remembered that these signs individually are of no importance, but if there are several that apply – sufficient to prevent the child from progressing normally – then they could be significant.

Reading and Spelling

Confusion of letters similar in shape: *d, b; u, n*.

Confusion of letters similar in sound: *d, t*; short vowels.

Reversals: was, saw.

Transposals: left, felt; auction, caution.

Omission or insertion of words.

Repetition or words or phase.

Changing sequence of words: she is, is she; stick walking, walking stick.

Confusion of small word: of, for, from.

Bizarre spelling.

Reading

Difficulty in keeping correct place on line.

Difficulty in switching from end of line to beginning of next one.

Mispronouncing even familiar words: skabetti – spaghetti.

Faulty auditory sequencing; emeny, enemy; hostipal, hospital.

No expression, or intonation in wrong place.

Difficulty in understanding a passage even if correctly read.

If the reader looks away from the page, he will be slow in finding his place again.

Writing

Bizarre spelling.

Foreshortening: rember, remember; sudly, suddenly.

Repetition of word or words.

Captials left out or in the wrong places.

i's not dotted, *t*'s not crossed, *l*'s crossed.

Badly formed letters or, if shape is correct, formed in unconventional way – even though correct formation has been taught.

Difficulty in keeping writing on the line.

Omission of punctuation, confusion over punctuation and syntax.

Odd pencil grip.

Difficulty in copying from blackboard.

Other Indications

Confusion between; right, left; east, west; up, down; etc

Difficulty in sequencing: alphabet, days, months of the year or numbers, words in sequence, telephone numbers.

Difficulty in learning tables.

Slow in looking up words in a dictionary, or names in a telephone directory.

Poor concentration, tires quickly.

Holds pen too tightly so whole arm aches.

Difficulty in interpreting other symbols: figures, notes in music, morse, etc.

Late learning to speak.

Late in learning to tell time and in such things as tying shoe laces, etc.

Other bad spellers in the family, including the extended family.

Difficulty in copying from blackboard.

Difficulty in finding the word he wants when speaking or writing.

Generally rather disorganised.

General Considerations

A point which is not always appreciated is the fatigue suffered by the struggling child. He has to put more effort into every aspect of reading and writing than his contemporaries do and, as reading or writing comes into almost every school subject, this puts him under a constant strain. After his first year or two at school he is always in a hurry trying to keep up and trying to manage, through conscious effort, a mass of small problems and details which by now come automatically to his peers. As he writes his thoughts may go something like this; "... Which way does a d go? ...Should that word have had a capital?... Which letter comes first in the word who?... Was there a full stop?... Why did I put a capital in the middle of that word?" ...Uncertainty is always present, nagging in the background: "...Is that word spelt right or is it not?..." Many a properly spelt word has been 'corrected' and made wrong because of this uncertainty.

Similar pressures may be present in reading. Even after a dyslexic has learned to read with apparent proficiency, he may still do so slowly, inaccurately or with poor comprehension. A passage may have to be read two or three or even four times before it can be fully understood.

Associations relating to symbols do not seem to form readily for the group under discussion. They may know the shapes and names of many letters, but the link that pairs the right two together is slow to form. Similarly a word may look like just a group of letters which need sorting out, and the meaning is not inherent in the look of the whole word. A digit may not be associated with the number it represents. Notes printed on a page will not suggest the musical tone, and punctuation marks do not indicate a pause or a change in the inflection of the voice. So many things which become automatic for most children have to be laboriously learned by the dyslexic.

If a reader, not already conversant with specific learning difficulty, has read as far as this he may well feel that this difficulty is a total disaster and with so many problems the only solution is to give up altogether. But this is not the case at all. Having worked in this field for many years I have seen so many young people go out into the world, many of them with their difficulties not fully understood, and make a great success of their lives. Some of those who have done brilliantly have already been mentioned.

The explanation is probably to be found in a combination of factors. The power of compensation is staggering. In addition, the dyslexic uses his good intelligence to find ways round any problem. With encouragement he develops remarkable persistence and ingenuity in overcoming weaknesses. This very persistence and staying power is a valuable lesson learnt. When faced with a problem later in life, he is often better able to face up to and tackle a difficulty than his peers whose academic successes have come more easily.

Dyslexia may be found at any intelligence level. However, those with low I.Q.s are rarely seen to be dyslexic as their failures are due mainly to their limited abilities.

A diagnosis of dyslexia (whatever term is used) may come as a shock to some parents, but the more they learn about it the less anxious they feel.

Learning the reason for a dismal school record is the first important step in restoring the confidence which is so vital in tackling a problem. When a child sees that all his efforts result in failure, he is almost certain sooner or later to give up the unequal struggle. But if the reason for his failure is identified and it can be explained to him why he has failed, his enemy is no longer abstract and unbeatable but something he can perhaps get to grips with. With this realisation and the necessary help comes the possibility of success, and with it the incentive to renew his efforts.

I shall never forget my own feelings when in my early twenties I was told that I was dyslexic. Feelings of hopelessness gradually turned to elation as the full meaning slowly sank in. Perhaps I was not stupid after all!